The

Vegan Cookbook

2021

Ultimate Cookbook with Vegan
Recipes for Happiness. Easy and
Tasty Vegan Food for you and the
Whole Family

Augustine Johns

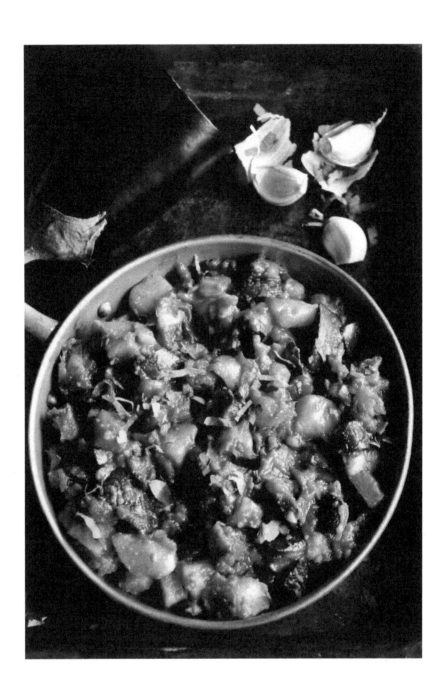

Table of Contents

The information in the following pages is broadly considered a truthful and accurate account of facts and as such, any inattention, use, or misuse of the information in question by the reader will render any resulting actions solely under their purview. There are no scenarios in which the publisher or the original author of this work can be in any fashion deemed liable for any hardship or damages that may befall them after undertaking information described herein.

Additionally, the information in the following pages is intended only for informational purposes and should thus be thought of as universal. As befitting its nature, it is presented without assurance regarding its prolonged validity or interim quality. Trademarks that are mentioned are done without written consent and can in no way be considered an endorsement from the trademark holder.

INTRODUCTION

The Merriam Webster Dictionary defines a vegetarian as one contains a wholly of vegetables, grains, nuts, fruits, and sometimes eggs or dairy products. It has also been described as a plant-based diet that relies wholly on plant-foods such as fruits, whole grains, herbs, vegetables, nuts, seeds, and spices. Whatever way you want to look at it, the reliance wholly on plants stands the vegetarian diet out from other types of diets. People become vegetarians for different reasons. Some take up this nutritional plan for medical or health reasons. For example, people suffering from cardiovascular diseases or who stand the risk of developing such diseases are usually advised to refrain from meat generally and focus on a plant-based diet, rich in fruits and vegetables. Some other individuals become vegetarians for religious or ethical reasons.

On this side of the spectrum are Hinduism, Jainism, Buddhism, Seventh-Day Adventists, and some other religions. It is believed that being a vegetarian is part of being holy and keeping with the ideals of non-violence. For ethical reasons, some animal rights activists are also vegetarians based on the belief that animals have rights and should not be slaughtered for food. Yet another set of persons become vegetarians based on food preference. Such individuals are naturally more disposed to a plant-based diet and find meat and other related food products less pleasurable. Some refrain from meat as a protest against climate change. This is based on the environmental concern that rearing livestock contributes to climate change and greenhouse gas emissions and the waste of natural resources in maintaining such livestock. People are usually very quick to throw words around without exactly knowing what a Vegetarian Diet means. In the same vein, the term "vegetarian" has become a popular one in recent years. What exactly does this word connote, and what does it not mean?

At its simplest, the word "vegetarian" refers to a person who refrains from eating meat, beef, pork, lard, chicken, or even fish. Depending on the kind of vegetarian it is, however, a vegetarian could either eat or exclude from his diet animal products. Animal products would refer to foods such as eggs, dairy products, and even honey! A vegetarian diet would, therefore, refer to the nutritional plan of the void of meat. It is the eating lifestyle of individuals who depend on plant-based foods for nutrition. It excludes animal products, particularly meat - a common denominator for all kinds of Vegetarians - from their diets. A vegetarian could also be defined as a meal plan that consists of foods coming majorly from plants to the exclusion of meat, poultry, and seafood.

This kind of Vegetarian diet usually contains no animal protein.

It is completely understandable from the discussion so far that the term "vegetarian" is more or less a blanket term covering different plant-based diets. While reliance majorly on plant foods is consistent in all the different types of vegetarians, they have some underlying differences. The different types of vegetarians are discussed below:

Veganism: This is undoubtedly the strictest type of vegetarian diet. Vegans exclude the any animal product. It goes as far as avoiding animal-derived ingredients contained in processed foods. Whether its meat, poultry products like eggs, dairy products inclusive of milk, honey, or even gelatin, they all are excluded from the vegans.

Some vegans go beyond nutrition and go as far as refusing to wear clothes that contain animal products. This means such vegans do not wear leather, wool, or silk.

Lacto-vegetarian: This kind of vegetarian excludes meat, fish, and poultry. However, it allows the inclusion of dairy products such as milk, yogurt, cheese, and butter. The hint is perhaps in the name since Lacto means milk in Latin.

Ovo-Vegetarian: Meat and dairy products are excluded under this diet, but eggs could be consumed. Ovo means egg.

Lacto-Ovo Vegetarian: This appears to be the hybrid of the Ovo Vegetarian and the Lacto-Vegetarian. This is the most famous type of vegetarian diet and is usually what comes to mind when people think of the Vegetarian. This type of Vegetarian bars all kinds of meat but allows for the consumption of eggs and dairy products.

Pollotarian: This vegetarian allows the consumption of chicken.

Pescatarian: This refers to the vegetarian that consumes fish. More people are beginning to subscribe to this kind of diet due to health reasons.

Flexitarian: Flexitarians are individuals who prefer plant-based foods to meat but have no problem eating meats once in a while. They are also referred to as semi-vegetarians.

Raw Vegan: This is also called the raw food and consists of a vegan that is yet to be processed and has also not been heated over 46 C. This kind of diet has its root in the belief that nutrients and minerals present in the plant diet are lost when cooked on temperature above 46 C and could also become harmful to the body.

White Bean and Artichoke Sandwich

Preparation Time: 15 minutes

Cooking Time: 10 minutes

Servings: 4

Ingredients:

- 1 ¼ cooked white beans
- ½ cup cashew nuts
- 6 artichoke hearts, chopped
- ¼ cup sunflower seeds, hulled
- 1 clove of garlic, peeled
- ¼ teaspoon salt
- ¼ teaspoon ground black pepper
- 1 teaspoon dried rosemary
- 1 lemon, grated
- 6 tablespoons almond milk, unsweetened
- 8 pieces of rustic bread

Directions:

1. Soak cashew nuts in warm water for 10 minutes, then drain them and transfer into a food processor.

2. Add garlic, salt, black pepper, rosemary, lemon zest, and milk and then pulse for 2 minutes until smooth, scraping the sides of the container frequently.
3. Take a medium bowl, place beans in it, mash them by using a fork, then add sunflower seeds and artichokes and stir until mixed.
4. Pour in cashew nuts dressing, stir until coated, and taste to adjust seasoning.
5. Take a medium skillet pan, place it over medium heat, add bread slices, and cook for 3 minutes per side until toasted.
6. Spread white beans mixture on one side of four bread slices and then cover with the other four slices.
7. Serve straight away.

Nutrition: 220 Cal 8 g Fat 1 g Saturated Fat 28 g Carbohydrates 8 g Fiber 2 g Sugars 12 g Protein;

Egg Salad Sandwich

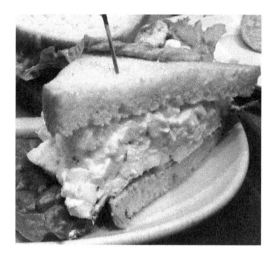

Preparation Time: 5 minutes

Cooking Time: 0 minutes

Servings: 4

Ingredients:

- 12 ounces tofu, extra-firm, pressed, drained
- 4 tablespoon sliced green onion
- ¼ teaspoon ground black pepper
- ½ teaspoon black salt
- 1/8 teaspoon turmeric powder
- 1 teaspoon mustard powder
- 8 teaspoons pumpkin seeds, shelled
- 4 tablespoon mayonnaise

- 8 slices of sandwich bread

Directions:

1. Take a medium bowl, place tofu in it, and then crumble it by using fingers.
2. Add remaining ingredients except for bread and stir until well combined, taste to adjust seasoning.
3. Take a medium skillet pan, place it over medium heat, add bread slices, and cook for 3 minutes per side until toasted.
4. Spread tofu mixture on one side of four bread slices and then cover with the other four slices.
5. Serve straight away.

Nutrition: 347 Cal 17 g Fat 2 g Saturated Fat 32 g Carbohydrates 2 g Fiber 4 g Sugars 15 g Protein;

Sabich Sandwich

Preparation Time: 10 minutes

Cooking Time: 10 minutes

Servings: 4

Ingredients:

- 1/2 cup cooked white beans
- 2 medium potatoes, peeled, boiled, ½-inch thick sliced
- 1 medium eggplant, destemmed, ½-inch cubed
- 4 dill pickles, ¼-inch thick sliced
- ¼ teaspoon of sea salt
- 2 tablespoons olive oil
- 1/4 teaspoon harissa paste
- 1/2 cup hummus
- 1 tablespoon mayonnaise
- 4 pita bread pockets
- 1/2 cup tabbouleh salad

Directions:

1. Take a small frying pan, place it over medium-low heat, add oil and wait until it gets hot.

17

2. Season eggplant pieces with salt, add to the hot frying pan and cook for 8 minutes until softened, and when done, remove the pan from heat.

3. Take a small bowl, place white beans in it, add harissa paste and mayonnaise and then stir until combined.

4. Assemble the sandwich and for this, place pita bread on clean working space, smear generously with hummus, then cover half of each pita bread with potato slices and top with a dill pickle slices.

5. Spoon 2 tablespoons of white bean mixture on each dill pickle, top with 3 tablespoons of cooked eggplant pieces and 2 tablespoons of tabbouleh salad and then cover the filling with the other half of pita bread.

6. Serve straight away.

Nutrition: 386 Cal 13 g Fat 2 g Saturated Fat 56 g Carbohydrates 7 g Fiber 3 g Sugars 12 g Protein;

Tofu and Pesto Sandwich

Preparation Time: 10 minutes

Cooking Time: 15 minutes

Servings: 4

Ingredients:

- 2 blocks of tofu, firm, pressed, drain
- 8 slices of tomato
- 8 leaves of lettuce
- 1 ½ teaspoon dried oregano
- ½ cup green pesto
- 2 tablespoons olive oil
- 8 slices of sandwich bread

Directions:

1. Switch on the oven, then set it to 375 degrees F and let it preheat.
2. Cut tofu into thick slices, place them in a baking sheet, drizzle with oil and sprinkle with oregano, and bake the tofu pieces for 15 minutes until roasted.
3. Assemble the sandwich and for this, spread pesto on one side of each bread slice, then top

four slices with lettuce, tomato slices, and roasted tofu and then cover with the other four slices.

4. Serve straight away.

Nutrition: 277 Cal 9.1 g Fat 1.5 g Saturated Fat 33.1 g Carbohydrates 3.6 g Fiber 12.7 g Sugars 16.1 g Protein;

Chickpea and Mayonnaise Salad Sandwich

Preparation Time: 10 minutes

Cooking Time: 0 minutes

Servings: 4

Ingredients:

For the mayonnaise:

- 1/3 cup cashew nuts, soaked in boiling water for 10 minutes
- ½ teaspoon ground black pepper
- 1 teaspoon salt
- 6 teaspoons apple cider vinegar
- 2 teaspoon maple syrup
- 1/2 teaspoon Dijon mustard

For the chickpea salad:

- 1 small bunch of chives, chopped
- 1 ½ cup sweetcorn
- 3 cups cooked chickpeas

To serve:

- 4 sandwich bread
- 4 leaves of lettuce

- ½ cup chopped cherry tomatoes

Directions:

1. Prepare the mayonnaise and for this, place all of its ingredients in a food processor and then pulse for 2 minutes until smooth, scraping the sides of the container frequently.
2. Take a medium bowl, place chickpeas in it, and then mash by using a fork until broken.
3. Add chives and corn, stir until mixed, then add mayonnaise and stir until well combined.
4. Assemble the sandwich and for this, stuff sandwich bread with chickpea salad, top each sandwich with a lettuce leaf, and ¼ cup of chopped tomatoes and then serve.

Nutrition: 387 Cal 19 g Fat 5 g Saturated Fat 39.7 g Carbohydrates 7.2 g Fiber 4.6 g Sugars 10 g Protein;

Mushrooms Sandwich

Preparation Time: 10 minutes

Cooking Time: 5 minutes

Servings: 4

Ingredients:

- 8 cherry tomatoes, halved
- 2 ounces of baby spinach
- 20 ounces of oyster mushrooms
- 2/3 teaspoon salt
- 1/3 teaspoon ground black pepper
- 2 tablespoons olive oil
- 4 tablespoons of barbecue sauce
- 8 slices of bread, toasted

Directions:

1. Take a griddle pan, place it over medium-high heat, grease it with oil and let it preheat.
2. Cut mushroom into thin strips, add to the hot griddle pan, drizzle with oil and cook for 5 minutes until done.

3. Transfer grilled mushrooms into a medium bowl, season with salt and black pepper, add barbecue sauce and toss until mixed.

4. Spread prepared mushroom mixture evenly on four bread slices, top with spinach and cherry tomatoes, then cover with the other four slices and serve.

Nutrition: 350 Cal 11 g Fat 3 g Saturated Fat 46 g Carbohydrates 9 g Fiber 7.2 g Sugars 12.1 g Protein;

Jalapeno Rice Noodles

Preparation Time: 10 minutes

Cooking Time: 25 minutes

Servings: 4

Ingredients

- ¼ cup soy sauce
- 1 tablespoon brown sugar
- 2 teaspoons sriracha
- 3 tablespoons lime juice
- 8 oz. rice noodles
- 3 teaspoons toasted sesame oil
- 1 package extra-firm tofu, pressed
- 1 onion, sliced
- 2 cups green cabbage, shredded
- 1 small jalapeno, minced
- 1 red bell pepper, sliced
- 1 yellow bell pepper, sliced
- 3 garlic cloves, minced
- 3 scallions, sliced
- 1 cup Thai basil leaves, roughly chopped
- Lime wedges for serving

Directions:

1. Fill a suitably-sized pot with salted water and boil it on high heat.
2. Add pasta to the boiling water and cook until it is al dente, then rinse under cold water.
3. Put lime juice, soy sauce, sriracha, and brown sugar in a bowl then mix well.
4. Place a large wok over medium heat then add 1 teaspoon sesame oil.
5. Toss in tofu and stir for 5 minutes until golden-brown.
6. Transfer the golden-brown tofu to a plate and add 2 teaspoons oil to the wok.
7. Stir in scallions, garlic, peppers, cabbage, and onion.
8. Sauté for 2 minutes, then add cooked noodles and prepared sauce.
9. Cook for 2 minutes, then garnish with lime wedges and basil leaves.
10. Serve fresh.

Nutrition: Calories: 45 Fat: 2.5g Protein: 4g Carbohydrates: 9g Fiber: 4g Sugar: 3g Sodium: 20mg

Rainbow Soba Noodles

Preparation Time: 10 minutes

Cooking Time: 20 minutes

Servings: 4

Ingredients

- 8 oz. tofu, pressed and crumbled
- 1 teaspoon olive oil
- ½ teaspoon red pepper flakes
- 10 oz. package buckwheat soba noodles, cooked
- 1 package broccoli slaw
- 2 cups cabbage, shredded
- ¼ cup very red onion, thinly sliced
- Peanut Sauce
- ¼ cup peanut butter
- ¾ cup hot water
- 2 tablespoons apple cider vinegar
- 1 tablespoon maple syrup
- 1–2 garlic cloves, minced
- 1 lime, zest, and juice
- Salt and crushed red pepper flakes, to taste
- Cilantro, for garnish

- Crushed peanuts, for garnish

Directions:

1. Crumble tofu on a baking sheet and toss in 1 teaspoon oil and 1 teaspoon red pepper flakes.

2. Bake the tofu for 20 minutes at 400°F in a preheated oven.

3. Meanwhile, whisk peanut butter with hot water, garlic cloves, maple syrup, cider vinegar, lime zest, salt, lime juice, and pepper flakes in a large bowl.

4. Toss in cooked noodles, broccoli slaw, cabbages, and onion.

5. Mix well, then stir in tofu, cilantro, and peanuts.

6. Enjoy.

Nutrition: Calories: 45 Fat: 2.5g Protein: 4g Carbohydrates: 9g Fiber: 4g Sugar: 3g Sodium: 20mg

Spicy Pad Thai Pasta

Preparation Time: 10 minutes

Cooking Time: 10 minutes

Servings: 4

Ingredients

- Spicy Tofu
- 1 lb. extra-firm tofu, sliced
- 1 tablespoon peanut butter
- 3 tablespoons soy sauce
- 2 tablespoons Sriracha
- 2 tablespoons rice vinegar
- 2 teaspoons sesame oil
- 2 teaspoons ginger, grated
- Pad Thai
- 8 oz. brown rice noodles
- 2 teaspoons coconut oil
- 1 red pepper, sliced
- ½ white onion, sliced
- 2 carrots, sliced
- 1 Thai chili, chopped
- ½ cup peanuts, chopped
- ½ cup cilantro, chopped

- Spicy Pad Thai Sauce
- 3 tablespoons soy sauce
- 3 tablespoons fresh lime juice
- 1 tablespoon Sriracha
- 3 tablespoons brown sugar
- 3 tablespoons vegetable broth
- 1 teaspoon garlic-chili paste
- 2 garlic cloves, minced

Directions:

1. Fill a suitably-sized pot with water and soak rice noodles in it.
2. Press the tofu to squeeze excess liquid out of it.
3. Place a non-stick pan over medium-high heat and add tofu.
4. Sear the tofu for 2-3 minutes per side until brown.
5. Whisk all the ingredients for tofu crumbles in a large bowl.
6. Stir in tofu and mix well.
7. Separately mix the pad Thai sauce in a bowl and add to the tofu.
8. Place a wok over medium heat and add 1 teaspoon oil.

9. Toss in chili, carrots, onion, and red pepper, then sauté for 3 minutes.

10. Transfer the veggies to the tofu bowl.

11. Add more oil to the same pan and stir in drained noodles, then stir cook for 1 minute.

12. Transfer the noodles to the tofu and toss it all well.

13. Add cilantro and peanuts.

14. Serve fresh.

Nutrition: Calories: 45 Fat: 2.5g Protein: 4g Carbohydrates: 9g Fiber: 4g Sugar: 3g Sodium: 20mg

Linguine with Wine Sauce

Preparation Time: 10 minutes

Cooking Time: 18 minutes

Servings: 4

Ingredients:

- 1 tablespoon olive oil
- 5 garlic cloves, minced
- 16 oz. shiitake, chopped
- ¼ teaspoon salt
- ¼ teaspoon ground pepper
- 1 pinch red pepper flakes
- ½ cup dry white wine
- 12 oz. linguine
- 2 teaspoons vegan butter
- ¼ cup Italian parsley, finely chopped

Directions:

1. Fill a suitably-sized pot with salted water and bring it to a boil on high heat.
2. Add pasta to the boiling water then cook until it is al dente, then rinse under cold water.

3. Place a non-stick skillet over medium-high heat then add olive oil.

4. Stir in garlic and sauté for 1 minute.

5. Stir in mushrooms and cook for 10 minutes.

6. Add salt, red pepper flakes, and black pepper for seasoning.

7. Toss in the cooked pasta and mix well.

8. Garnish with parsley and butter.

9. Enjoy.

Nutrition: Calories: 40; Fat: 2.0g Protein: 5g

Carbohydrates: 7g Fiber: 4g Sugar: 3g

Cheesy Macaroni with Broccoli

Preparation Time: 10 minutes

Cooking Time: 25 minutes

Servings: 6

Ingredients

- 1/3 cup melted coconut oil
- ¼ cup nutritional yeast
- 1 tablespoon tomato paste
- 1 tablespoon dried mustard
- 2 garlic cloves, minced
- 1 ½ teaspoons salt
- ½ teaspoon ground turmeric
- 4 ½ cups almond milk
- 3 cups cauliflower florets, chopped
- 1 cup raw cashews, chopped
- 1 lb. shell pasta
- 1 tablespoon white vinegar
- 3 cups broccoli florets

Directions:

1. Place a suitably-sized saucepan over medium heat and add coconut oil.

2. Stir in mustard, yeast, garlic, salt, tomato paste, and turmeric.
3. Cook for 1 minute then add almond milk, cashews, and cauliflower florets.
4. Continue cooking for 20 minutes on a simmer.
5. Transfer the cauliflower mixture to a blender jug then blend until smooth.
6. Stir in vinegar and blend until creamy.
7. Fill a suitably-sized pot with salted water and bring it to a boil on high heat.
8. Add pasta to the boiling water.
9. Place a steamer basket over the boiling water and add broccoli to the basket.
10. Cook until the pasta is al dente. Drain and rinse the pasta and transfer the broccoli to a bowl.
11. Add the cooked pasta to the cauliflower-cashews sauce.
12. Toss in broccoli florets, salt, and black pepper.
13. Mix well then serve.

Nutrition: Calories: 40; Fat: 2.0g Protein: 5g Carbohydrates: 7g Fiber: 4g Sugar: 3g Sodium: 18mg

Soba Noodles with Tofu

Preparation Time: 10 minutes

Cooking Time: 38 minutes

Servings: 4

Ingredients

- Marinated Tofu
- 2 tablespoons olive oil
- 8 oz. firm tofu, pressed and drained
- ¼ cup cilantro, finely chopped
- ¼ cup mint, finely chopped
- 1-inch fresh ginger, grated
- Soba Noodles
- 8 oz. soba noodles
- ¾ cup edamame
- 2 cucumbers, peeled and julienned
- 1 large carrot, peeled and julienned
- 2 tablespoons black sesame seeds
- 2 tablespoons white sesame seeds
- 2 scallions, chopped
- Ginger-Soy Sauce
- 2 tablespoons fresh lime juice
- 2 tablespoons soy sauce

- 1 tablespoon brown sugar
- 1 tablespoon fresh ginger, grated
- 2 tablespoons sesame oil
- ½ tablespoon garlic chili sauce

Directions:

1. Blend herbs, ginger, salt, black pepper, and olive oil in a blender.
2. Add the spice mixture to the tofu and toss it well to coat.
3. Allow the tofu to marinate for 30 minutes at room temperature.
4. Fill a suitably-sized pot with salted water and bring it to a boil on high heat.
5. Add pasta to the boiling water then cook until it is al dente, then rinse under cold water.
6. Place a large wok over medium heat and add marinated tofu.
7. Sauté for 5–8 minutes until golden-brown, then transfer to a large bowl.
8. Add veggies to the same wok and stir until veggies are soft.
9. Transfer the veggies to the tofu and add cooked noodles.

10.Toss well, then serve warm.

11.Enjoy.

Nutrition: Calories: 30; Fat: 3.5.0g Protein: 6g

Carbohydrates: 6g Fiber: 4g; Sugar: 5g Sodium:

18mg

Plant Based Keto Lo Mein

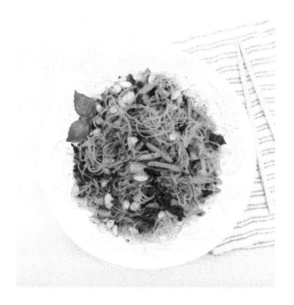

Preparation Time: 10 minutes

Cooking Time: 10 minutes

Servings: 2

Ingredients:

- 2 tablespoons carrots, shredded

- 1 package kelp noodles, soaked in water

- 1 cup broccoli, frozen

- For the Sauce

- 1 tablespoon sesame oil

- 2 tablespoons tamari

- ½ teaspoon ground ginger
- ¼ teaspoon Sriracha
- ½ teaspoon garlic powder

Directions:

1. Put the broccoli in a saucepan on medium low heat and add the sauce ingredients.
2. Cook for about 5 minutes and add the noodles after draining water.
3. Allow to simmer about 10 minutes, occasionally stirring to avoid burning.
4. When the noodles have softened, mix everything well and dish out to serve.

Nutrition: Calories: 30; Fat: 3.5.0g Protein: 6g Carbohydrates: 6g Fiber: 4g;

Vegetarian Chow Mein

Preparation Time: 20 minutes

Cooking Time: 30 minutes

Servings: 2

Ingredients:

- ½ large onion, chopped
- ½ small leek, chopped
- ½ tablespoon ginger paste
- ½ tablespoon Worcester sauce
- ½ tablespoon Oriental seasoning
- ½ teaspoon parsley
- Salt and black pepper, to taste
- ½ pound noodles
- 2 large carrots, diced
- 2 celery sticks, chopped
- 1 tablespoon olive oil
- ½ teaspoon garlic paste
- 1½ tablespoons soy sauce
- 1 tablespoon Chinese five spice
- ½ teaspoon coriander
- 2 cups water

Directions:

1. Put olive oil, ginger, garlic paste, and onion in a pot on medium heat and sauté for about 5 minutes.
2. Stir in all the vegetables and cook for about5 minutes.
3. Add rest of the ingredients and combine well.
4. Secure the lid and cook on medium heat for about 20 minutes, stirring occasionally.
5. Open the lid and dish out to serve hot.

Nutrition: Calories: 30; Fat: 3.5.0g Protein: 6g Carbohydrates: 6g Fiber: 4g; Sugar: 5g Sodium: 18mg

Veggie Noodles

Preparation Time: 10 minutes

Cooking Time: 5 minutes

Servings: 2

Ingredients:

- 2 tablespoons vegetable oil
- 4 spring onions, divided
- 1 cup snap pea
- 2 tablespoons brown sugar
- 9 oz. dried rice noodles, cooked
- 5 garlic cloves, minced
- 2 carrots, cut into small sticks
- 3 tablespoons soy sauce

Directions:

1. Heat vegetable oil in a skillet over medium heat and add garlic and 3 spring onions.
2. Cook for about 3 minutes and add the carrots, peas, brown sugar and soy sauce.
3. Add rice noodles and cook for about 2 minutes.
4. Season with salt and black pepper and top with remaining spring onion to serve.

Nutrition: Calories: 25; Fat: 2.0g Protein: 5.2g

Carbohydrates: 5.3g Fiber: 4g; Sodium: 18mg

Minutes Vegetarian Pasta

Preparation Time: 5 minutes

Cooking Time: 16 minutes

Servings: 4

Ingredients:

- 3 shallots, chopped
- ¼ teaspoon red pepper flakes
- ¼ cup vegan parmesan cheese
- 2 tablespoons olive oil
- 2 garlic cloves, minced
- 8-ounces spinach leaves
- 8-ounces linguine pasta
- 1 pinch salt
- 1 pinch black pepper

Directions:

1. Boil salted water in a large pot and add pasta.
2. Cook for about 6 minutes and drain the pasta in a colander.
3. Heat olive oil over medium heat in a large skillet and add the shallots.

4. Cook for about 5 minutes until soft and caramelized and stir in the spinach, garlic, red pepper flakes, salt and black pepper.

5. Cook for about 5 minutes and add pasta and 2 ladles of pasta water.

6. Stir in the parmesan cheese and dish out in a bowl to serve.

Nutrition: Calories: 25; Fat: 2.0g Protein: 5.2g Carbohydrates: 5.3g Fiber: 4g; Sodium: 18mg

Pesto Quinoa with White Beans

Preparation Time: 5 minutes

Cooking Time: 15 minutes

Servings: 4

Ingredients:

- 12 ounces cooked white bean
- 3 ½ cups quinoa, cooked
- 1 medium zucchini, sliced
- ¾ cup sun-dried tomato
- ¼ cup pine nuts
- 1 tablespoon olive oil

For the Pesto:

- 1/3 cup walnuts
- 2 cups arugula
- 1 teaspoon minced garlic
- 2 cups basil
- ¾ teaspoon salt
- ¼ teaspoon ground black pepper
- 1 tablespoon lemon juice
- 1/3 cup olive oil
- 2 tablespoons water

Directions:

1. Prepare the pesto, and for this, place all of its ingredients in a food processor and pulse for 2 minutes until smooth, scraping the sides of the container frequently and set aside until required.

2. Take a large skillet pan, place it over medium heat, add oil and when hot, add zucchini and cook for 4 minutes until tender-crisp.

3. Season zucchini with salt and black pepper, cook for 2 minutes until lightly brown, then add tomatoes and white beans and continue cooking for 4 minutes until white beans begin to crisp.

4. Stir in pine nuts, cook for 2 minutes until toasted, then remove the pan from heat and transfer zucchini mixture into a medium bowl.

5. Add quinoa and pesto, stir until well combined, then distribute among four bowls and then serve.

Nutrition: 352 Cal 27.3 g Fat 5 g Saturated Fat 33.7 g Carbohydrates 5.7 g Fiber 4.5 g Sugars 9.7 g Protein;

Green Bean Casserole

Preparation Time: 5 minutes

Cooking Time: 40 minutes

Servings: 4

Ingredients:

- 6 ounces fried onions
- 1 ½ cups cremini mushrooms, diced
- 16 ounces frozen green beans
- ½ cup diced white onion
- 1 tablespoon minced garlic
- 3 ½ tablespoons all-purpose flour
- 1/3 teaspoon ground black pepper
- ½ teaspoon dried oregano
- 3 ½ tablespoons olive oil
- 2 cups vegetable broth, hot

Directions:

1. Switch on the oven, then set it to 400 degrees F and let it preheat.
2. Take a medium saucepan, place it over medium heat, add oil and when hot, add onion and

mushrooms, stir in garlic and cook for 4 minutes until tender.

3. Stir in flour until the thick paste comes together and then cook for 2 minutes until golden.

4. Stir in vegetable broth, bring it to a simmer, then stir in black pepper and oregano, whisk well and cook for 15 minutes until gravy thickened to the desired level.

5. Add green beans, stir until mixed, remove the pan from heat, top beans with fried onions and bake for 15 minutes.

6. Serve straight away.

Nutrition: 191 Cal 10 g Fat 2 g Saturated Fat 22 g Carbohydrates 3.3 g Fiber 2.5 g Sugars 4.1 g Protein;

Pumpkin Risotto

Preparation Time: 5 minutes

Cooking Time: 20 minutes

Servings: 4

Ingredients:

- 1 cup Arborio rice
- ½ cup cooked and chopped pumpkin
- 1/2 cup mushrooms
- 1 rib of celery, diced
- ½ of a medium white onion, peeled, diced
- ½ teaspoon minced garlic
- ½ teaspoon salt
- 1/3 teaspoon ground black pepper
- 1 tablespoon olive oil
- ½ tablespoon coconut butter
- 1 cup pumpkin puree
- 2 cups vegetable stock

Directions:

1. Take a medium saucepan, place it over medium heat, add oil and when hot, add onion and

celery, stir in garlic and cook for 3 minutes until onions begin to soften.

2. Add mushrooms, season with salt and black pepper and cook for 5 minutes.

3. Add rice, pour in pumpkin puree, then gradually pour in the stock until rice soaked up all the liquid and have turned soft.

4. Add butter, remove the pan from heat, stir until creamy mixture comes together, and then serve.

Nutrition: 218.5 Cal 5.2 g Fat 1.5 g Saturated Fat 32.3 g Carbohydrates 1.3 g Fiber 3.8 g Sugars 6.3 g Protein;

Brown Rice and Vegetable Stir-Fry

Preparation Time: 5 minutes

Cooking Time: 50 minutes

Servings: 4

Ingredients:

- 16-ounce tofu, extra-firm, pressed, drained, cut into ½-inch cubes
- 1 cup of brown rice
- 1 cup frozen broccoli florets
- 1 medium red bell pepper, cored, diced
- 1 small white onion, peeled, diced
- 1 tablespoon minced garlic
- ½ teaspoon salt
- 1/3 teaspoon ground black pepper
- 1 tablespoon olive oil
- 2 cups vegetable broth

Directions:

1. Take a medium pot, place it over high heat, add brown rice, pour in vegetable broth, and bring it to a boil.

2. Switch heat to medium-low level, cover the pot with the lid and cook for 40 minutes, and when done, remove the pot and set aside until required.

3. Then take a large skillet pan, place it over medium-high heat, add oil and when hot, add tofu pieces, onion, broccoli, and bell pepper, season with salt and black pepper and cook for 5 minutes until sauté.

4. Add cooked rice, stir until mixed and continue cooking for 5 minutes.

5. Serve straight away.

Nutrition: 281.9 Cal 11.7 g Fat 1.7 g Saturated Fat 31.1 g Carbohydrates 9.7 g Fiber 2.1 g Sugars 20.1 g Protein;

Tomato Basil Spaghetti

Preparation Time: 5 minutes

Cooking Time: 20 minutes

Servings: 4

Ingredients:

- 15-ounce cooked great northern beans
- 10.5-ounces cherry tomatoes, halved
- 1 small white onion, peeled, diced
- 1 tablespoon minced garlic
- 8 basil leaves, chopped
- 2 tablespoons olive oil
- 1-pound spaghetti

Directions:

1. Take a large pot half full with salty water, place it over medium-high heat, bring it to a boil, add spaghetti and cook for 10 to 12 minutes until tender.

2. Then drain spaghetti into a colander and reserve 1 cup of pasta liquid.

3. Take a large skillet pan, place it over medium-high heat, add oil and when hot, add onion,

tomatoes, basil, and garlic and cook for 5
minutes until vegetables have turned tender.

4. Add cooked spaghetti and beans, pour in pasta
   water, stir until just mixed and cook for 2
   minutes until hot.

5. Serve straight away.

Nutrition: 147 Cal 5 g Fat 0.7 g Saturated Fat
21.2 g Carbohydrates 1.5 g Fiber 5.4 g Sugars 3.8
g Protein;

Jamaican Jerk Tofu Wrap

Preparation Time: 1 hour and 15 minutes

Cooking Time: 16 minutes

Servings: 4

Ingredients:

- 28 ounces tofu, firmed, pressed, drain, ½-inch long sliced

For the Marinade:

- 2 small scotch bonnet pepper, deseeded, minced
- 2 teaspoons minced garlic
- 2 1/2 teaspoons sea salt
- 4 teaspoons allspice
- 2 teaspoon ground black pepper
- 4 teaspoons cinnamon
- 4 teaspoons maple syrup
- 4 teaspoons nutmeg
- 4 tablespoons apple cider vinegar
- 2 teaspoon avocado oil and more for cooking
- ½ cup of soy sauce
- 2 tablespoon tomato paste

For the Wrap:

- 4 cups baby spinach leaves
- 2 small tomato, deseeded, diced
- 2 medium yellow bell pepper, deseeded, cut into strips
- 4 tablespoons Sriracha sauce
- 4 tortillas, whole-grain

Directions:

1. Take a large bowl, place all the ingredients for the marinade in it, whisk until combined, then add tofu pieces, toss until well coated, and let it marinate for a minimum of 1 hour, turning halfway.

2. Then take a large skillet pan, place it over medium-high heat, add some of the avocado oil, and when hot, add tofu pieces in a single layer and cook for 8 minutes per side until caramelized.

3. Assemble the wrap and for this, place a tortilla on clean working space, top with 1 cup of spinach, half of each diced tomatoes and pepper strips, then top with 4 strips of tofu, drizzle with Sriracha sauce and wrap tightly.

4. Repeat with the remaining tortilla, then cut each tortilla in half and serve.

Nutrition: 250 Cal 6 g Fat 1 g Saturated Fat 40 g Carbohydrates 7 g Fiber 11 g Sugars 9 g Protein;

Bean and Rice Burritos

Preparation Time: 10 minutes

Cooking Time: 20 minutes

Servings: 6

Ingredients:

- 32 ounces refried beans

- 2 cups cooked rice

- 2 cups chopped spinach

- 1 tablespoon olive oil

- 1/2 cup tomato salsa

- 6 tortillas, whole-grain, warm

- Guacamole as needed for serving

Directions:

1. Switch on the oven, then set it to 375 degrees F and let it preheat.

2. Take a medium saucepan, place it over medium heat, add beans, and cook for 3 to 5 minutes until softened, remove the pan from heat.

3. Place one tortilla on clean working space, spread some of the beans on it into a log, leaving 2-inches of the edge, top beans with spinach, rice

and salsa, and then tightly wrap the tortilla to seal the filling like a burrito.

4. Repeat with the remaining tortillas, place these burritos on a baking sheet, brush them with olive oil and then bake for 15 minutes until golden.

5. Serve burritos with guacamole.

Nutrition: 421 Cal 9 g Fat 2 g Saturated Fat 70 g Carbohydrates 11 g Fiber 3 g Sugars 15 g Protein;

Chickpea Curry Soup

Preparation Time: 5 minutes

Cooking Time: 12 minutes

Servings: 4

Ingredients:

- 2 cups cooked chickpeas
- 1/4 of a medium white onion, peeled, chopped
- 1 tablespoon minced garlic
- 1 teaspoon ground coriander
- ¼ teaspoon cayenne pepper
- 1 tablespoon yellow curry powder
- 1 teaspoon turmeric
- ½ of a lime, juiced
- 1 tablespoon olive oil
- 2/3 cup coconut cream
- 2 cups vegetable broth
- 2 tablespoons pumpkin seeds

Directions:

1. Take a medium saucepan, place it over medium-high heat, add oil and when hot, add onion and garlic and cook for 1 minute until fragrant.

2. Add chickpeas, sprinkle with all the spices, stir until mixed and continue cooking for 5 minutes.
3. Pour in vegetable broth, simmer for 5 minutes, then stir in cream, lime juice and remove the pan from heat.
4. Ladle soup into bowls, top with pumpkin seeds, and then serve.

Nutrition: 154 Cal 8 g Fat 1 g Saturated Fat 16.5 g Carbohydrates 4 g Fiber 3 g Sugars 4.5 g Protein;

Roasted Vegetables and Tofu Salad

Preparation Time: 10 minutes

Cooking Time: 25 minutes

Servings: 4

Ingredients:

- For the salad:
- 2 cups chopped tofu, firm, pressed, drained
- 2 cups cooked chickpeas
- 4 cups spinach
- 2 cups broccoli floret
- 2 cups chopped sweet potato, peeled
- 2 cups Brussel sprout, halved
- 4 teaspoons ground black pepper
- 4 teaspoons salt
- 4 tablespoons red chili powder
- 1 cup olive oil
- For the dressing:
- 2 teaspoons salt
- 2 teaspoons ground black pepper
- 4 teaspoons dried thyme

- 4 tablespoons lemon juice
- 4 tablespoons olive oil
- 2 teaspoons water
- ½ cup hummus

Directions:

1. Switch on the oven, then set it to 400 degrees F and let it preheat.

2. Take a large baking sheet, grease it with oil, and spread broccoli florets in one-fifth of the portion, reserving few florets for later use.

3. Add sprouts, sweet potatoes, tofu, and chickpeas as an individual pile on the baking sheet, drizzle with oil, season with salt, black pepper, and red chili powder and then bake for 25 minutes until the tofu has turned nicely golden brown and vegetables are softened, tossing halfway.

4. While vegetables, grains, and tofu are being roasted, prepare the dressing and for this, take a medium jar, add all of its ingredients in it, stir until well combined, and then divide the dressing among four large mason jars.

5. When vegetables, grains, and tofu has been roasted, distribute evenly among four mason jars along with reserved cauliflower florets and shut with lid.

6. When ready to eat, shake the Mason jar until salad is coated with the dressing and then serve.

Nutrition: 477 Cal 24 g Fat 5 g Saturated Fat 52 g Carbohydrates 16 g Fiber 11 g Sugars 21 g Protein;

Farro and Lentil Salad

Preparation Time: 10 minutes

Cooking Time: 0 minutes

Servings: 4

Ingredients:

For the Salad:

- 1 cup grape tomato, halved
- ½ cup diced yellow bell pepper
- 1 cup diced cucumber,
- ½ cup diced red bell pepper
- 1 cup fresh arugula
- 1/3 cup chopped parsley
- 1 ½ cups lentils, cooked
- 3 ½ cups farro, cooked

For the Dressing:

- ½ teaspoon minced garlic
- ½ teaspoon salt
- ¼ teaspoon ground black pepper
- 1 teaspoon Italian seasoning
- 1 teaspoon Dijon mustard
- 2 tablespoons red wine vinegar

- 2 tablespoons lemon juice
- 1/3 cup olive oil

Directions:

1. Take a large bowl, place all the ingredients for the salad in it except for arugula and then toss until combined.
2. Prepare the dressing and for this, take a medium bowl, add all of its ingredients in it and then stir whisk until well combined.
3. Pour the dressing over the salad, toss until well coated, then distribute salad among four bowls and top with arugula.
4. Serve straight away.

Nutrition: 379 Cal 10 g Fat 2 g Saturated Fat 63.5 g Carbohydrates 11 g Fiber 2.5 g Sugars 12.5 g Protein;

Greek Zoodle Bowl

Preparation Time: 10 minutes

Cooking Time: 0 minutes

Servings: 4

Ingredients:

- ½ cup chopped artichokes
- 14 cherry tomatoes, chopped
- 1 medium red bell peppers, cored, chopped
- 4 medium zucchini
- 1 medium yellow bell pepper, cored, chopped
- 6 tablespoons hemp hearts
- 1 English cucumber
- 6 tablespoons chopped red onion
- 2 tablespoons chopped parsley leaves
- 2 tablespoons chopped mint

For the Greek Dressing:

- 2 tablespoons chopped mint
- 1 teaspoon garlic powder
- ½ teaspoon salt
- ¼ teaspoon dried oregano
- 2 teaspoons Italian seasoning

- 3 tablespoons red wine vinegar
- 1 tablespoon olive oil

Directions:

1. Prepare zucchini and cucumber noodles and for this, spiralize them by using a spiralizer or vegetable peeler and then divide evenly among four bowls.

2. Top zucchini and cucumber noodles with artichokes, tomato, bell pepper, hemp hearts, onion, parsley, and mint and then set aside until required.

3. Prepare the dressing and for this, take a small bowl, add all the ingredients for the dressing in it and whisk until combined.

4. Add the prepared dressing evenly into each bowl, then toss until the vegetables are well coated with the dressing and serve.

Nutrition: 250 Cal 14 g Fat 3 g Saturated Fat 19 g Carbohydrates 5 g Fiber 9 g Sugars 13 g Protein;

Roasted Vegetables and Quinoa Bowls

Preparation Time: 10 minutes

Cooking Time: 20 minutes

Servings: 4

Ingredients:

- 3 cups cooked quinoa

For the Broccoli:

- 2 teaspoons minced garlic
- 4 cups broccoli florets
- ½ teaspoon salt
- ¼ teaspoon ground black pepper
- 4 teaspoons olive oil

For the Chickpeas:

- 4 teaspoons sriracha
- 3 cups cooked chickpeas
- 2 teaspoons olive oil
- 4 teaspoons soy sauce

For the Roasted Sweet Potatoes:

- 2 teaspoons curry powder

- 2 small sweet potatoes, peeled, ¼-inch thick sliced
- 1/8 teaspoon salt
- 2 teaspoons sriracha
- 2 teaspoons olive oil

For the Chili-Lime Kale:

- 1/2 of a lime, juiced
- 4 cups chopped kale
- 1/8 teaspoon salt
- 1/8 teaspoon ground black pepper
- 1 teaspoon red chili powder
- 2 teaspoons olive oil

Directions:

1. Switch on the oven, then set it to 400 degrees F and let it preheat.
2. Prepare broccoli florets and for this, take a large bowl, place all of its ingredients in it, toss until well coated, then take a baking sheet lined with parchment paper and spread florets in a one-third portion of the sheet in a row.
3. Add chickpeas into the bowl, add its remaining ingredients, toss until well mixed and spread

them onto the baking sheet next to the broccoli florets.

4. Add sweet potatoes into the bowl, add its remaining ingredients, toss until well mixed and spread them onto the baking sheet next to the chickpeas.

5. Place the baking sheet containing vegetables and chickpeas into the oven and then bake for 20 minutes until vegetables have turned tender and chickpeas are slightly crispy, turning halfway.

6. Meanwhile, prepare the kale and for this, take a large skillet pan, place it over medium heat, add 1 teaspoon oil and when hot, add kale and cook for 5 minutes until tender.

7. Then season kale with salt, black pepper, and red chili powder, toss until mixed and continue cooking for 3 minutes, set aside until required.

8. Assemble the bowl and for this, distribute quinoa evenly among four bowls, top evenly with broccoli, chickpeas, sweet potatoes, and kale and then serve.

Nutrition: 415 Cal 17 g Fat 2 g Saturated Fat 54 g Carbohydrates 8 g Fiber 5 g Sugars 16 g Protein;

Sweet Potato and Quinoa Bowl

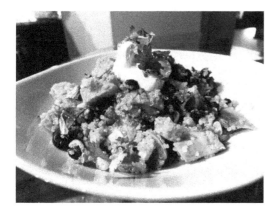

Preparation Time: 5 minutes

Cooking Time: 20 minutes

Servings: 4

Ingredients:

- 2 cups quinoa
- 1 cup diced red onion
- 2 cups diced sweet potato
- 1 1/2 cup raisins
- 1 cup sunflower seeds, shelled, unsalted
- 2 cups vegetable broth

Directions:

1. Take a medium pot, place it over high heat, add quinoa, and sweet potatoes, pour in vegetable broth, stir until mixed and bring it to a boil.
2. Then switch heat to medium-low level, cover pot with the lid, and cook for 20 minutes until the quinoa has cooked.
3. When done, remove the pot from heat and fluff quinoa by using a fork.
4. Add onion, raisins, and sunflower seeds, stir until mixed and transfer into a large bowl.
5. Let it chill in the refrigerator for 30 minutes and then serve.

Nutrition: 204 Cal 7 g Fat 3 g Saturated Fat 31 g Carbohydrates 3 g Fiber 11 g Sugars 3 g Protein;

Chickpea Salad Bites

Preparation Time: 15 minutes

Cooking Time: 0 minutes

Servings: 4

Ingredients:

For the Bread:

- 2 tablespoons chopped parsley
- 1 small green chili pepper
- 1/3 cup of raisins
- 1 teaspoon garlic powder
- ½ teaspoon salt
- 1/3 teaspoon ground black pepper
- ½ teaspoon smoked paprika
- ½ tablespoon maple syrup
- ½ teaspoon cayenne pepper
- 2 tablespoons balsamic vinegar
- 1 1/2 cups crumbled rye bread, whole-grain

For the Salad:

- 2 scallions, chopped
- 1/3 cup chopped pickles

- 2 tablespoons chopped chives and more for topping
- ½ teaspoon minced garlic
- 1 ½ cup cooked chickpeas
- 1 lemon, juiced
- ½ teaspoon salt
- ¼ teaspoon ground black pepper
- 1 tablespoons poppy seeds
- 1 teaspoon mustard paste
- 1/3 cup coconut yogurt

Directions:

1. Prepare the bread, and for this, place all of its ingredients in a food processor and then pulse for 1 minute until just combined; don't overmix.

2. Then make bites of the bread mixture and for this, take a 2.3-inch round cookie cutter, add 2 tablespoons of the bread mixture, press it into the cutter, and gently lift it out, repeat with the remaining batter to make seven more bites.

3. Prepare the salad and for this, take a large bowl, add chickpeas in it, then add chives, scallion, pickles, and garlic and then mash chickpeas by using a fork until broken.

4. Add remaining ingredients for the salad and stir until well mixed.

5. Assemble the bites and for this, top each prepared bread bite generously with prepared salad, sprinkle with chives and poppy seeds, and then serve.

Nutrition: 210 Cal 4 g Fat 1 g Saturated Fat 36 g Carbohydrates 6 g Fiber 4 g Sugars 7 g Protein;

Avocado and Chickpeas Lettuce Cups

Preparation Time: 10 minutes

Cooking Time: 0 minutes

Servings: 4

Ingredients:

- 2 small avocados, peeled, pitted, diced
- 8 ounces hearts of palm
- ¾ cup cooked chickpeas
- 1/2 cup cucumber, diced
- 1 tablespoon minced shallots
- 2 cups mixed greens
- 1 tablespoon Dijon mustard
- 1 lime, zested, juiced
- 2 tablespoons chopped cilantro and more for topping
- 2/3 teaspoon salt
- 1/3 teaspoon ground black pepper
- 1 tablespoon apple cider vinegar
- 2 ½ tablespoons olive oil

Directions:

1. Take a medium bowl, add shallots and cilantro in it, stir in salt, black pepper, mustard, vinegar, lime juice, and zest until just mixed and then slowly mix in olive oil until combined.
2. Add cucumber, hearts of palm and chickpeas, stir until mixed, fold in avocado and then top with some more cilantro.
3. Distribute mixed greens among four plates, top with chickpea mixture and then serve.

Nutrition: 280 Cal 12.6 g Fat 1.5 g Saturated Fat 32.8 g Carbohydrates 9.3 g Fiber 1.2 g Sugars 7.6 g Protein;

DINNER RECIPES

Glazed Avocado

Preparation Time: 10 minutes

Cooking Time: 12 minutes

Servings: 4

Ingredients:

- 1 tablespoon stevia
- 1 teaspoon olive oil
- 1 teaspoon water
- 1 teaspoon lemon juice
- ½ teaspoon rosemary, dried
- ½ teaspoon ground black pepper
- 2 avocados, peeled, pitted and cut into large pieces

Directions:

1. Heat up a pan with the oil over medium heat, add the avocados, stevia and the other ingredients, toss, cook for 12 minutes, divide into bowls and serve.

Nutrition: Calories 262 Fat 9.6 Fiber 0.1 Carbs 6.5 Protein 7.9

Mango and Leeks Meatballs

Preparation Time: 20 minutes

Cooking Time: 10 minutes

Servings: 4

Ingredients:

- 1 tablespoon mango puree
- 1 cup leeks, chopped
- ½ cup tofu, crumbled
- 1 teaspoon dried oregano
- 1 tablespoon almond flour
- 1 teaspoon olive oil
- 1 tablespoon flax meal
- ½ teaspoon chili flakes

Directions:

1. In the mixing bowl, mix up mango puree with leeks, tofu and the other ingredients except the oil and stir well.
2. Make the small meatballs.
3. After this, pour the olive oil in the skillet and heat it up.

4. Add the meatballs in the skillet and cook them for 4 minutes from each side.

Nutrition: Calories 147 Fat 8.6 Fiber 4.5 Carbs 5.6 Protein 5.3

Spicy Carrots and Olives

Preparation Time: 15 minutes

Cooking Time: 10 minutes

Servings: 4

Ingredients:

- ½ teaspoon hot paprika
- 1 red chili pepper, minced
- ¼ teaspoon ground cumin
- ¼ teaspoon dried oregano
- ¼ teaspoon dried basil
- ½ teaspoon salt
- 1 tablespoon olive oil
- 1 pound baby carrots, peeled
- 1 cup kalamata olives, pitted and halved
- juice of 1 lime

Directions:

1. Heat up a pan with the oil over medium heat, add the carrots, olives and the other ingredients, toss, cook for 10 minutes, divide between plates and serve.

Nutrition: Calories 141 Fat 5.8 Fiber 4.3 Carbs 7.5 Protein 9.6

Harissa Mushrooms

Preparation Time: 15 minutes

Cooking Time: 30 minutes

Servings: 4

Ingredients:

- 1-pound mushroom caps
- 1 teaspoon harissa
- 1 teaspoon rosemary, dried
- 2 spring onions, chopped
- 1 leek, sliced
- 1 teaspoon thyme, dried
- 1 cup crushed tomatoes
- 1 teaspoon sweet paprika
- A pinch of salt and black pepper
- 1 tablespoon olive oil
- ½ teaspoon lemon juice

Directions:

1. In a roasting pan, mix the mushrooms with the harissa, rosemary and the other ingredients and toss.
2. Preheat the oven to 360F and put the pan inside.

3. Cook the mix for 30 minutes, divide between plates and serve.

Nutrition: Calories 250 Fat 12.1 Fiber 5.3 Carbs 14.5 Protein 12.9

Leeks and Artichokes Mix

Preparation Time: 10 minutes

Cooking Time: 30 minutes

Servings: 4

Ingredients:

- 2 cups canned artichoke hearts, drained and quartered
- 3 leeks, sliced
- 1 cup cherry tomatoes, halved
- ¼ cup coconut cream
- 1 tablespoon almond flakes
- 1 teaspoon olive oil
- 1 teaspoon oregano, dried
- 1 teaspoon salt
- 1 teaspoon ground black pepper
- ¼ cup of chives, chopped

Directions:

1. Heat up a pan with the oil over medium heat, add the leeks, oregano, salt and pepper, stir and cook for 10 minutes.

2. Add artichokes and the other ingredients, toss, cook for 20 minutes, divide into bowls and serve.

Nutrition: Calories 234 Fat 9.7 Fiber 4.2 Carbs 9.6 Protein 12.3

Coconut Avocado

Preparation Time: 10 minutes

Cooking Time: 0 minutes

Servings: 2

Ingredients:

- 2 avocados, halved, pitted and roughly cubed
- 1 teaspoon dried thyme
- 2 tablespoons coconut cream
- 1 cup spring onions, chopped
- 1 teaspoon turmeric powder
- Salt and black pepper to the taste
- ¼ teaspoon cayenne pepper
- ½ teaspoon onion powder
- ½ teaspoon garlic powder
- 1 teaspoon paprika
- Salt and black pepper to the taste
- 2 tablespoons lemon juice

Directions:

1. In a bowl, mix the avocados with the thyme, coconut cream and the other ingredients, toss, divide between plates and serve.

Nutrition: Calories 160 Fat 6.9 Fiber 7 Carbs 12

Protein 7

Avocado Cream

Preparation Time: 10 minutes

Cooking Time: 0 minutes

Servings: 4

Ingredients:

- 2 avocados, pitted, peeled and chopped
- 3 cups veggie stock
- 1 teaspoon curry powder
- 1 teaspoon cumin, ground
- 1 teaspoon basil, dried
- 2 scallions, chopped
- Salt and black pepper to the taste
- 2 tablespoons coconut oil
- 2/3 cup coconut cream, unsweetened

Directions:

1. In a blender, mix the avocados with the stock, curry powder and the other ingredients, blend and serve.

Nutrition: Calories 212 Fat 8 Fiber 4 Carbs 6.1 Protein 4.1

Tamarind Avocado Bowls

Preparation Time: 10 minutes

Cooking Time: 0 minutes

Servings: 2

Ingredients:

- 1 teaspoon cumin seeds
- 1 tablespoon olive oil
- ½ teaspoon gram masala
- 1 teaspoon ground ginger
- 2 avocados, peeled, pitted and roughly cubed
- 1 mango, peeled, and cubed
- 1 cup cherry tomatoes, halved
- ½ teaspoon cayenne pepper
- 1 teaspoon turmeric powder
- 3 tablespoons tamarind paste

Directions:

1. In a bowl, mix the avocados with the mango and the other ingredients, toss and serve.

Nutrition: Calories 170 Fat 4.5 Fiber 3 Carbs 5 Protein 6

Onion and Tomato Bowls

Preparation Time: 10 minutes

Cooking Time: 0 minutes

Servings: 4

Ingredients:

- 1 tablespoon olive oil
- 2 red bell peppers, cut into thin strips
- 2 red onions, cut into thin strips
- Salt and black pepper to the taste
- 1 teaspoon dried basil
- 1 pound tomatoes, cut into wedges
- 1 teaspoon balsamic vinegar
- 1 teaspoon sweet paprika

Directions:

1. In a bowl, mix the peppers with the onions and the other ingredients, toss and serve.

Nutrition: Calories 107 Fat 4.5 Fiber 2 Carbs 7.1 Protein 6

Avocado and Leeks Mix

Preparation Time: 10 minutes

Cooking Time: 0 minutes

Servings: 4

Ingredients:

- 1 small red onion, chopped
- 2 avocados, pitted, peeled and chopped
- 1 teaspoon chili powder
- 2 leeks, sliced
- 1 cup cucumber, cubed
- 1 cup cherry tomatoes, halved
- Salt and black pepper to the taste
- 2 tablespoons cumin powder
- 2 tablespoons lime juice
- 1 tablespoon parsley, chopped

Directions:

1. In a bowl, mix the onion with the avocados, chili powder and the other ingredients, toss and serve.

Nutrition: Calories 120 Fat 2 Fiber 2 Carbs 7 Protein 4

Lemon Lentils and Carrots

Preparation Time: 10 minutes

Cooking Time: 20 minutes

Servings: 6

Ingredients:

- 1 cup brown lentils, soaked overnight and drained
- 1 cup carrots, shredded
- 1 cup spring onions, chopped
- 1 teaspoon curry powder
- 1 teaspoon turmeric powder
- 1 teaspoon garam masala
- 2 tablespoons lemon juice
- ¼ cup parsley, chopped
- 2 garlic cloves, minced
- A pinch of salt and black pepper
- ½ teaspoon thyme, dried
- 2 tablespoons olive oil

Directions:

1. Heat up a pan with the oil over medium heat, add the garlic, carrots and spring onions and cook for 5 minutes.
2. Add the lentils and the other ingredients, toss and simmer over medium heat for 15 minutes.
3. Divide between plates and serve.

Nutrition: Calories 240 Fat 7 Fiber 3.4 Carbs 12 Protein 6

Cabbage Bowls

Preparation Time: 10 minutes

Cooking Time: 10 minutes

Servings: 4

Ingredients:

- 1 green cabbage head, shredded
- 1 red cabbage head, shredded
- 1 teaspoon garam masala
- 1 teaspoon basil, dried
- 1 teaspoon coriander, ground
- 1 teaspoon mustard seeds
- 1 tablespoon balsamic vinegar
- ¼ cup tomatoes, crushed
- A pinch of salt and black pepper
- 3 carrots, shredded
- 1 yellow bell pepper, chopped
- 1 orange bell pepper, chopped
- 1 red bell pepper, chopped
- 2 tablespoons dill, chopped
- 2 tablespoons olive oil

Directions:

1. Heat up a pan with the oil over medium heat, add the peppers and carrots and cook for 2 minutes.
2. Add the cabbage and the other ingredients, toss, cook for 10 minutes, divide between plates and serve.

Nutrition: Calories 150 Fat 9 Fiber 4 Carbs 3.3 Protein 4.4

Pomegranate and Pears Salad

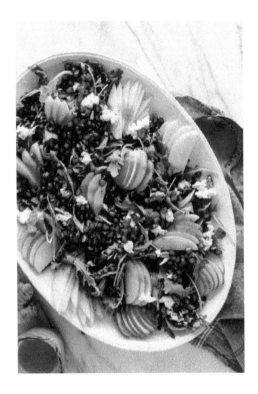

Preparation Time: 10 minutes

Cooking Time: 0 minutes

Servings: 3

Ingredients:

- 3 big pears, cored and cut with a spiralizer
- ¾ cup pomegranate seeds
- 2 cups baby spinach
- ½ cup black olives, pitted and cubed

- ¾ cup walnuts, chopped1 tablespoon olive oil
- 1 tablespoon coconut sugar
- 1 teaspoon white sesame seeds
- 2 tablespoons chives, chopped
- 1 tablespoon balsamic vinegar
- 1 garlic clove, minced
- A pinch of sea salt and black pepper

Directions:

1. In a bowl, mix the pears with the pomegranate seeds, spinach and the other ingredients, toss and serve.

Nutrition: Calories 200 Fat 3.9 Fiber 4 Carbs 6 Protein 3.3

Bulgur and Tomato Mix

Preparation Time: 15 minutes

Cooking Time: 0 minutes

Servings: 4

Ingredients:

- 1 ½ cups hot water
- 1 cup bulgur
- Juice of 1 lime
- 1 cup cherry tomatoes, halved
- 4 tablespoons cilantro, chopped
- ½ cup cranberries, dried
- juice of ½ lemon
- 1 teaspoon oregano, dried
- 1/3 cup almonds, sliced
- ¼ cup green onions, chopped
- ½ cup red bell peppers, chopped
- ½ cup carrots, grated
- 1 tablespoon avocado oil
- A pinch of sea salt and black pepper

Directions:

1. Place bulgur into a bowl, add boiling water to it, stir, and cover and set aside for 15 minutes.
2. Fluff bulgur with a fork and transfer to a bowl.
3. Add the rest of the ingredients, toss and serve.

Nutrition: Calories 260 Fat 4.4 Fiber 3 Carbs 7 Protein 10

Beans Mix

Preparation Time: 10 minutes

Cooking Time: 15 minutes

Servings: 4

Ingredients:

- 1 ½ cups cooked black beans
- 1 cup cooked red kidney beans
- ½ teaspoon garlic powder
- ½ teaspoon smoked paprika
- 2 teaspoons chili powder
- 1 tablespoon olive oil
- 1 ½ cups chickpeas, cooked
- 1 teaspoon garam masala
- 1 red bell pepper, chopped
- 2 tomatoes, chopped
- 1 cup cashews, chopped
- ½ cup veggie stock
- 1 tablespoon balsamic vinegar
- 1 tablespoon oregano, chopped
- 1 tablespoon dill, chopped
- 1 cup corn kernels, chopped

Directions:

1. Heat up a pan with the oil over medium heat, add the beans, garlic powder, chili powder and the other ingredients, toss and cook for 15 minutes.
2. Divide between plates and serve.

Nutrition: Calories 300 Fat 8.3 Fiber 3.3 Carbs 6 Protein 13

Black Bean Burgers

Preparation Time: 10 minutes

Cooking Time: 15 minutes

Servings: 6

Ingredients:

- 1 Onion, diced
- ½ cup Corn Nibs
- 2 Cloves Garlic, minced
- ½ teaspoon Oregano, dried
- ½ cup Flour
- 1 Jalapeno Pepper, small
- 2 cups Black Beans, mashed & canned
- ¼ cup Breadcrumbs (Vegan)
- 2 teaspoons Parsley, minced
- ¼ teaspoon cumin
- 1 tablespoon Olive Oil
- 2 teaspoons Chili Powder
- ½ Red Pepper, diced
- Sea Salt to taste

Directions:

1. Set your flour on a plate, and then get out your garlic, onion, peppers and oregano, throwing it in a pan. Cook over medium-high heat, and then cook until the onions are translucent. Place the peppers in, and sauté until tender.
2. Cook for two minutes, and then set it to the side.
3. Use a potato masher to mash your black beans, then stir in the vegetables, cumin, breadcrumbs, parsley, salt, and chili powder, and then divide it into six patties.
4. Coat each side, and then cook until it is fried on each side.

Nutrition: Calories: 357 kcal Protein: 17.93 g Fat: 5.14 g Carbohydrates: 61.64 g

Dijon Maple Burgers

Preparation Time: 20 minutes

Cooking Time: 30 minutes

Servings: 12

Ingredients:

- 1 Red Bell Pepper
- 19 ounces Can Chickpeas, rinsed & drained
- 1 cup Almonds, ground
- 2 teaspoons Dijon Mustard
- 1 teaspoon Oregano
- ½ teaspoon Sage
- 1 cup Spinach, fresh
- 1 – ½ cups Rolled Oats
- 1 Clove Garlic, pressed
- ½ Lemon, juiced
- 2 teaspoons Maple Syrup, pure

Directions:

1. Get out a baking sheet. Line it with parchment paper.
2. Cut your red pepper in half and then take the seeds out. Place it on your baking sheet, and

roast in the oven while you prepare your other ingredients.

3. Process your chickpeas, almonds, mustard, and maple syrup together in a food processor.

4. Add in your lemon juice, oregano, sage, garlic, and spinach, processing again. Make sure it's combined, but don't puree it.

5. Once your red bell pepper is softened, which should roughly take ten minutes, add this to the processor as well. Add in your oats, mixing well.

6. Form twelve patties, cooking in the oven for a half-hour. They should be browned.

Nutrition: Calories: 96 kcal Protein: 5.28 g Fat: 2.42 g Carbohydrates: 16.82 g

Hearty Black Lentil Curry

Preparation Time: 30 minutes

Cooking Time: 6 hours and 15 minutes

Servings: 4

Ingredients:

- 1 cup of black lentils, rinsed and soaked overnight
- 14 ounce of chopped tomatoes
- 2 large white onions, peeled and sliced
- 1 1/2 teaspoon of minced garlic
- 1 teaspoon of grated ginger
- 1 red chili
- 1 teaspoon of salt
- 1/4 teaspoon of red chili powder
- 1 teaspoon of paprika
- 1 teaspoon of ground turmeric
- 2 teaspoons of ground cumin
- 2 teaspoons of ground coriander
- 1/2 cup of chopped coriander
- 4-ounce of vegetarian butter
- 4 fluid of ounce water
- 2 fluid of ounce vegetarian double cream

Directions:

1. Place a large pan over moderate heat, add butter and let heat until melt.

2. Add the onion and garlic and ginger and cook for
   - 10 to 15 minutes or until onions are caramelized.

3. Then stir in salt, red chili powder, paprika, turmeric, cumin, ground coriander, and water.

4. Transfer this mixture to a 6-quarts slow cooker and add tomatoes and red chili.

5. Drain lentils, add to slow cooker, and stir until just mix.

6. Plugin slow cooker; adjust cooking time to 6 hours and let cook on low heat setting.

7. When the lentils are done, stir in cream and adjust the seasoning.

8. Serve with boiled rice or whole wheat bread.

Nutrition: Calories: 299 kcal Protein: 5.59 g Fat: 27.92 g Carbohydrates: 9.83 g

Flavorful Refried Beans

Preparation Time: 15 minutes

Cooking Time: 8 hours

Servings: 8

Ingredients:

- 3 cups of pinto beans, rinsed
- 1 small jalapeno pepper, seeded and chopped
- 1 medium-sized white onion, peeled and sliced
- 2 tablespoons of minced garlic
- 5 teaspoons of salt
- 2 teaspoons of ground black pepper
- 1/4 teaspoon of ground cumin
- 9 cups of water

Directions:

1. Using a 6-quarts slow cooker, place all the ingredients and stir until it mixes properly.
2. Cover the top, plug in the slow cooker, adjust the cooking time to 6 hours, let it cook on the high heat setting, and add more water if the beans get too dry.

3. When the beans are done, drain it then reserve the liquid.

4. Mash the beans using a potato masher and pour in the reserved cooking liquid until it reaches your desired mixture.

5. Serve immediately.

Nutrition: Calories: 268 kcal Protein: 16.55 g Fat: 1.7 g Carbohydrates: 46.68 g

Conclusion

Vegan recipes do not need to be boring. There are so many different combinations of veggies, fruits, whole grains, beans, seeds, and nuts that you will be able to make unique meal plans for many months. These recipes contain the instructions along with the necessary ingredients and nutritional information.

If you ever come across someone complaining that they can't follow the plant-based diet because it's expensive, hard to cater for, lacking in variety, or tasteless, feel free to have them take a look at this book. In no time, you'll have another companion walking beside you on this road to healthier eating and better living.

Although healthy, many people are still hesitant to give vegan food a try. They mistakenly believe that these would be boring, tasteless, and complicated to make. This is the farthest thing from the truth.

Fruits and vegetables are organically delicious, fragrant, and vibrantly colored. If you add herbs, mushrooms, and nuts to the mix, dishes will always come out packed full of flavor it only takes a bit of effort and time to prepare great-tasting vegan meals for your family.

How easy was that? Don't we all want a seamless and easy way to cook like this?

I believe cooking is taking a better turn and the days, when we needed so many ingredients to provide a decent meal, were gone. Now, with easy tweaks, we can make delicious, quick, and easy meals. Most importantly, we get to save a bunch of cash on groceries.

I am grateful for downloading this book and taking the time to read it. I know that you have learned a lot and you had a great time reading it. Writing books is the best way to share the skills I have with your and the best tips too.

I know that there are many books and choosing my book is amazing. I am thankful that you stopped and took time to decide. You made a great decision and I am sure that you enjoyed it.

I will be even happier if you will add some comments. Feedbacks helped by growing and they still do. They help me to choose better content and new ideas. So, maybe your feedback can trigger an idea for my next book.

Hopefully, this book has helped you understand that vegetarian recipes and diet can improve your life, not only by improving your health and helping you lose weight, but also by saving you money and time. I sincerely hope that the recipes provided in this book have proven to be quick, easy, and delicious, and have provided you with enough variety to keep your taste buds interested and curious.

I hope you enjoyed reading about my book!